Hives, Headaches & Heartburn

Heal Your Histamine Hangover

H_2N ... NH ... N

by

Beverley Rider,
PhD, NC

ISBN: 978-1-7329072-2-5

Library of Congress #:2019915672

Copyright 2019 by Beverley Rider, PhD NC

For more information, visit www.rider4health.org.

Summerland Publishing, 3181 E. Elgin Drive, Salt Lake City, UT 84109.

Printed in the United States of America.

Layout and Cover Design by Pizzirani Consulting, Summerland, CA. Contact: pizziraniconsulting@yahoo.com

Kind Words

- ♥ A sincere thank you to Dr. Ed Bauman for guiding me through writing this book and through rocky times.

- ♥ A warm thank you to Dr. Samuel Yanuck for his scientific review.

- ♥ A huge thank you to Stacey Hutson and Jolinda Pizzirani for their endless edits and clever wordsmithing.

- ♥ A heartfelt thank you to my friends (Marion, April, and Kate) for encouraging me to write this.

- ♥ A loving thank you to my family (Alfred, Margaret, David, Janette, and Paul) for being supportive and patient with me.

- ♥ A loving thank you to my now healthy teenage daughter, Tayla, who started her life with illness. She inspired me to dive into the evidence on puzzling reactions and to want to help others, too.

Dedication

To you, reader: I truly hope that sharing our healing journey will help you in yours.

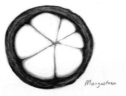

Mangosteen

A portion of proceeds from this book will be donated to charities involved in understanding and relieving histamine and mast cell illness.

Details can be found online at *Rider4Health.org*.

She was six days old, and there we were in the ER at 3 AM. My daughter was having a reaction. To what? And why? They had no answers. EKGs and blood tests confirmed that she was fine. But just twenty minutes earlier, her airway was blocked with a sticky mass that even paramedics weren't able to clear. It was the scariest night of my life.

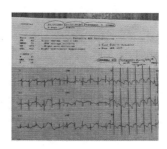

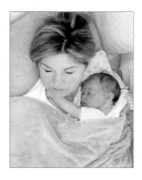

She survived the night, but her life was followed by years of reactions with hives, headaches, heartburn, and other puzzling complaints, and one too many days off from school. Not to mention the anxiety and embarrassment she suffered as a result.

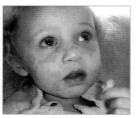

However, all the standard allergy and other testing came up negative. I felt helpless. Humbled. Here I was with a PhD in immunology, working as a biotech scientist, and I couldn't understand what was going on with my own daughter's immune system. Even my husband, an MD, was at a loss. Was it all in our heads?

That's when I turned to integrative medicine. With the support of a few incredible practitioners, we were able to get to the root of the problem and help my daughter heal her body and enjoy her childhood. She went from being an anxious little girl to a confident young teen, completing her first triathlon at eight years old. I, too, had changed. Once I discovered integrative medicine, I couldn't go back to my old career. Instead, I followed my research and passion to Bauman College to earn my certification in Nutrition.

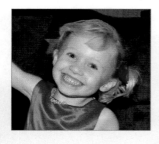

I am eternally grateful for all the integrative healers who have come before me. The following pages briefly summarize my years of research, client consulting, and personal experience. My hope is that after you read 'Hives, Headaches, and Heartburn: Heal Your Histamine Hangover,' you will find answers too.

Table of Contents

Meet David — the chronic allergy sufferer

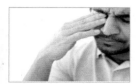

"My eyes are itchy and red almost all the time. My nose is runny, sinuses hurt, and I'm constantly blocked up. I can't sleep at night because I can't breathe. Feels like an ongoing cold, but it can't be. It's really just the norm for me now. I can never leave home without my antihistamines."

Meet Amanda — with the never-ending migraine

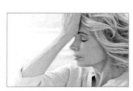

"You'll often find me in my office, lights off, fingers pressed into my temples. I feel lucky if I catch a day without my head throbbing, but they are few and far between. People ask me if I'm hungover. Ironically, I don't drink much anymore. I just don't have the tolerance I used to. I've ditched red wine, chocolate and cheese altogether because they make it worse. I feel like I'm eating all the right things, yet I constantly feel anxious, irritable, and overwhelmed from the ongoing achy pain like a nail driven into my head. Oh, and the brain fog!

Meet Betty — bloated with every bite

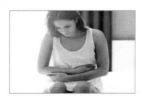

"After I eat, my belly gets big and bloated. I'm a second grade teacher, and one of my students asked me if I was pregnant. Ouch! I get so gassy that when I walk, I let out little toots with each footstep. Nausea, burping, diarrhea, you name it, I've got it. I worry about going out and not finding a bathroom in time. I feel like I spend half my time on the toilet, hoping to get some relief."

David, Amanda, and Betty have something in common. They have an overload of histamine wreaking havoc on their bodies. You may have heard of histamine and antihistamine, but there's a lot more to it that meets the itchy eye.

Their individual symptoms may seem very different because excess histamine is exerting its effect on different systems in their bodies. For David, it's his respiratory system. For Amanda, it's her nervous system. And for Betty, it's her digestive system.

Histamine excess, also called histamine intolerance (HIT), is underdiagnosed and surprisingly common, and affects many people in many different ways. If some of these symptoms apply to you, read on.

Common Symptoms of Histamine Excess

Airway/Allergy
- runny nose/congestion
- sneezing
- red, itchy, watery eyes
- sore throat, cough
- asthma-like symptoms
- food reactions

Digestion
- diarrhea
- stomachaches/cramps
- bloating/flatulence
- reflux/heartburn
- nausea/vomiting

Skin
- itchiness
- hives/eczema/other rashes
- reaction to insect bites
- swelling, especially facial

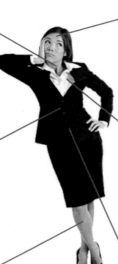

Nervous System
- headache/migraine
- dizziness/vertigo
- insomnia
- mood swings/anxiety
- motion/sea/car sickness

Cardiovascular
- blood pressure changes
- dizziness and fainting
- rapid heartbeat/palpitations
- low blood pressure

Other
- menstrual cycle issues, PMS
- joint and muscle pain
- multiple confusing symptoms
- extreme fatigue

Read on for odd or unusual symptoms

---

4 Reasons to Balance Histamine

1. Histamine is metabolically greedy meaning it uses up a lot of nutrients and taxes the liver and body in general.

2. It causes inflammation in the body, which makes you feel miserable.

3. Excess histamine can be dangerous at high levels.

4. Many of the causes of imbalance can be healed naturally.

What is Histamine? What are Mast Cells?

Histamine isn't the enemy, but an important chemical messenger secreted by mast cells and other cells in response to inflammatory triggers such as infections or allergies. Mast cells produce and store histamine. They are found mostly in tissues throughout the body that are in contact with the external environment such as the mouth, nose, skin, lungs, and gut—on guard and ready to dispatch their histamine and other immune mediators if they detect danger.

In plain English? A mast cell is like a yippy chihuahua, and histamine is like his bark. If he senses danger, he becomes wary, his ears perk up, and he sounds the alarm with his bark. Over time, he calms down. However, if the threat continues, the chihuahua doubles his efforts and barks even louder, alerting more chihuahuas and other guard dogs, such as other immune cells.

Sometimes, harmless things such as pollen, in the case of allergy, can trigger the alarm (barking). However, the solution is not to get rid of the alarm system or even plug your ears (i.e., taking an antihistamine), but to calm him down so that he doesn't overreact to things that are harmless.

Mast Cell

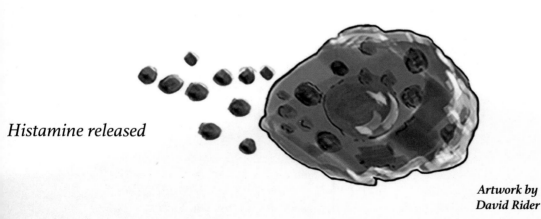

Histamine released

*Artwork by
David Rider*

How Does Histamine Work?

We all make histamine in our bodies and will all react given a high enough level. An example of this is a type of food poisoning called scombroid, which can occur after consuming spoiled fish. The fish contains dangerously high levels of histamine to which most people will react.

That's why the term Histamine Intolerant (HIT) can be confusing. You can be intolerant to lactose in dairy. But you can't be intolerant to something your body produces. It's not whether you can or can't tolerate histamine; it's how much you can tolerate. This boils down to the balance between histamine coming IN (via all sources of histamine) to histamine going OUT (and the capacity to remove it). Therefore, it would be more accurate to say Histamine "Excess" or "Overload." That said, to stay consistent with published studies, we'll stick with "Histamine Intolerant" (HIT).

In 1966, Dr. Carl Pfeiffer discovered that most people with schizophrenia had abnormal levels of histamine. He coined the terms "histadelia" (meaning high histamine) and "histapenia" (low histamine). As their levels were restored to normal, subjects experienced improvement in symptoms. Since Pfeiffer's discovery, researchers have found histamine imbalance doesn't stop at schizophrenia but can also drive anxiety, insomnia, acid reflux, sea sickness, eczema, small intestine bacterial overgrowth (SIBO), and migraines.

> *Histamine isn't all bad. It's crucial for our bodies to digest, think and defend. However, excess histamine can wreak havoc, causing different effects in different people.*

Main Causes of Excess Histamine

The accumulation of histamine is not usually noticed until levels exceed a threshold. Think of it as a bucket. Once full, any added histamine will cause it to overflow, flooding our system and causing a cascade of reactions.

The main causes of excess histamine include:

1. **Gene Expression**

2. **Immune Reaction:** Allergies, infections, and other substances that trigger mast cells

3. **Poor gut health:** due to infection, damage, antibiotics, or chemicals

4. **Diet:** Inflammatory and high histamine foods. These get the most press but are not usually the root cause. However, a reaction to these foods likely indicates an underlying imbalance that needs to be addressed

5. **Lifestyle:** Stress, lack of sleep, and medications, to name a few

6. **Imbalances in nutrients or hormones**

7. **Environment:** Mold, smoke, pesticides, EMF, and harsh chemicals

8. **Medications**

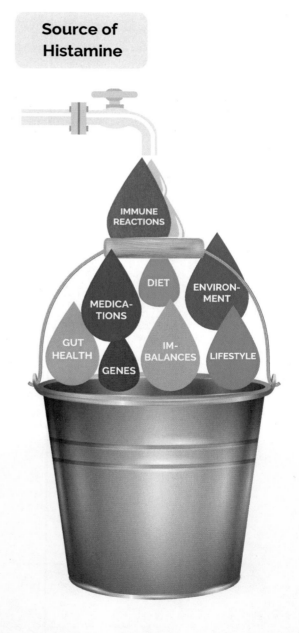

Source of Histamine

IMMUNE REACTIONS

DIET

ENVIRON-MENT

MEDICA-TIONS

GUT HEALTH

IM-BALANCES

LIFESTYLE

GENES

What Prevents Histamine Excess?

Specific enzymes degrade histamine to protect us from overload. One of the main enzymes is diamine oxidase (DAO), but many people lack adequate DAO for various reasons, and struggle to control excess histamine. How does inadequacy happen? The answer may be due to your genes, immune reactions, gut health (intestinal lining damage or unwanted bacteria growth), imbalances, diet (alcohol), lifestyle (stress), environment, or medications (ibuprofen). Less DAO activity means more histamine, so optimizing DAO is important.

Histamine N-Methyltransferase (HNMT) is a second enzyme that helps break down histamine on the inside of cells to prevent excess histamine.

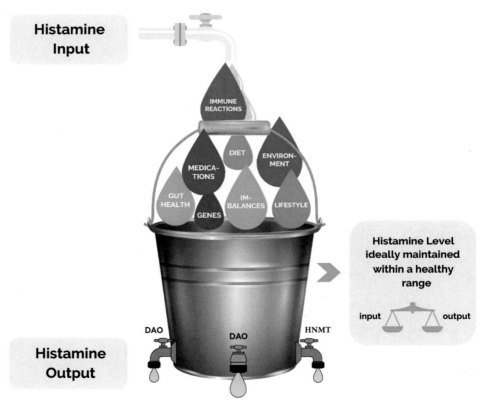

Symptoms Arise When
Histamine INPUT > Histamine OUTPUT

*Histamine intolerance occurs when your histamine
levels exceed your body's ability to remove it.*

Intolerance vs Allergy

There is a difference between an intolerance and an allergy. Acute food allergies, such as a peanut allergy, are relatively rare, well-characterized responses, mediated by a type of antibody called immunoglobulin E (IgE). They usually cause an immediate immune reaction every time a tiny amount of the specific allergen is encountered. Symptoms include sneezing, sniffling, itching, watery eyes, or perhaps hives, throat swelling, and (rarely) anaphylaxis.

In contrast, an intolerance such as lactose intolerance doesn't primarily involve the immune system; it involves the digestive system. A reaction can happen if your body lacks a specific ensyme such as lactase to break down lactose in milk. You may feel discomfort or downright miserable, but an intolerance is rarely life-threatening.

It's important to note, though, the two are not mutually exclusive. You can have allergies and react to histamine. However, if you react to histamine, you don't necessarily have a specific allergy. This means that histamine intolerance may not show up on your allergy test. As you can imagine, there is plenty of confusion surrounding these reactions. We do know that food allergies and HIT are distinct from each other, though their symptoms also greatly overlap.

> *Histamine excess and food allergies are distinct,*
> *but symptoms can overlap and be confused.*

Histamine Mechanism

Excess histamine can show up all over the body — as headaches, a runny nose, hives, and motion sickness, to name a few. Then there are the psychological effects like anxiety, moodiness, and insomnia. Regardless of symptoms, a healthy gut is not only vital for balancing histamine levels, but for overall health.

The Gut Brain Axis

Our gut has been called our "second brain." Why? Because it communicates with and affects the rest of our body, has nerve networks and even makes neurotransmitters. In fact, most of the body's serotonin is produced in the gut. So when the gut is inflamed, it can affect mood, sleep, memory, focus and so much more. It should be of no surprise, then, that histamine intolerance can develop in the gut.

Intestinal Permeability

Intestinal permeability, also called leaky gut, is a term that refers to the cells along the intestinal lining and how closely knit they are. Think of these cells as a border crossing between the intestine and the bloodstream. When this lining is healthy, the cells are close together, restricting access to the bloodstream.

The gut lining can become damaged or inflamed by poor diet, gut infections, medications, and imbalanced flora, leaving gaps between the cells. These gaps allow proteins, partially digested foods, bacteria and chemicals such as histamine to enter the bloodstream. Hence, the name, leaky gut.

Histamine in the Small Intestine / SIBO

Insufficient digestion can lead to reactions that trigger histamine. Therefore, people with gut-related conditions are at higher risk for HIT. Especially those with Small Intestinal Bacterial Overgrowth, more commonly known as SIBO. Research has shown that histamine is secreted when SIBO is active.

It's easy to understand how histamine is implicated in allergic conditions such as hay fever, asthma, and food allergies. But besides the immune system, histamine is also involved in every system of the body. This means HIT can contribute to vast non-allergic symptoms, too — conditions as diverse as menstrual pains, vertigo, seasickness, even psychological conditions like schizophrenia.

What does a reaction to histamine excess look like?

Consider an insect bite which triggers histamine release at the site. The tiny surrounding blood vessels then expand and become permeable, allowing immune cells and factors to leak into the area. Now the bite becomes swollen, red and itchy. In people with histamine excess, the bite may not stop at a small red spot but may grow into a huge raised, itchy bump. In fact, histamine itself notoriously causes itching, begging us to scratch. Problem is, the more we scratch, the more histamine gets released, causing more itchiness. While reactions of histamine on the skin are usually harmless, the entry of histamine into the bloodstream can be much more severe.

Not all of these symptoms will occur in any one person, and the severity of symptoms will increase with the levels and duration of histamine present in the body. Confusingly, many of these symptoms overlap with other illnesses, particularly allergies. This is because the body releases high levels of histamine during an allergic response. Given this overlap and the fact that HIT symptoms are so diverse, this condition can go undetected.

Symptoms can be acute or delayed, wax and wane, present differently one reaction to the next, and be quite strange. Dr. Ben Lynch even reported having excessively sweaty feet.

The clients that I typically see have felt chronically unwell for many years, have a long list of vague or strange symptoms, have consulted many practitioners, and often think it's all in their heads. They feel they are too weak, too complain-y, too highly sensitive, or even crazy. If this is you, I'm here to tell you that YOU ARE NOT! Give yourself a huge hug and know that if you suffer from excess histamine, you have been through more than some people ever will. Your symptoms may not always be visible or measurable, but they are very real, just as real as say, a broken arm.

The A-Ha moment for my clients usually comes when they: 1) see the patterns in their histamine triggers and 2) realize that histamine links their symptoms.

The Self-Test: Are you Histamine Intolerant?

Now that you understand better what histamine is and what it looks like, let's find out if you suffer from excess histamine. Check any of the following bullet points that you have experienced in the last 3 days, unless otherwise indicated. Note: This is not a diagnosis.

Allergy-like Responses

☐ Red, itchy, or watery eyes
☐ Sneezing, runny nose, or congestion
☐ Sensitive to certain foods (red wine, fermented foods, cheese, chocolate)
☐ Sensitive to certain smells, fumes or exhaust
☐ Coughing or frequent throat clearing
☐ Asthma or wheezing
☐ Known allergies

Digestive Responses

☐ Diarrhea or constipation (less common)
☐ Stomach cramps / abdominal pain
☐ Bloating
☐ Flatulence / gas
☐ Heartburn / acid reflux
☐ Upset stomach after eating
☐ Irritable Bowel Syndrome (IBS)
☐ Small Intestine Bacterial Overgrowth (SIBO)
☐ Nausea / vomiting

Skin Responses

☐ Itching
☐ Hives
☐ Rashes such as eczema or contact dermatitis
☐ Dark circles under eyes not due to lack of sleep
☐ Mouth / tongue sores
☐ Mouth itches or tingles after certain foods
☐ Reaction to insect bites, especially wasp (*hymenoptera*) stings
☐ Swelling, often around eyes and mouth
☐ Flushed red cheeks, ears, or nose
☐ Skin stays red long after being scratched
☐ React after sun exposure

Cardiovascular Responses

☐ Racing heart / fast heartbeat
☐ Heart pounding / heart palpitations
☐ Low blood pressure or sudden change in blood pressure
☐ Dizzy when standing up quickly
☐ Fainting

Nervous System and Psychological Responses

☐ Anxiety
☐ Rapid mood changes
☐ Depression
☐ Confusion / brain fog / poor focus
☐ Headaches
☐ Migraines
☐ Vertigo
☐ Insomnia
☐ Extreme fatigue
☐ Restless Leg Syndrome (RLS)
☐ Motion Sickness

Other Responses and Unusual Responses

☐ Premenstrual flare ups, PMS menstrual irregularities
☐ Joint and muscle pain / fibromyalgia
☐ Frequent bloody nose
☐ Sweaty hands and feet
☐ Ringing in ears

- ☐ Hot flashes
- ☐ Frequent urination or irritable bladder
- ☐ Excess salivation
- ☐ Weight gain or weight cycling
- ☐ Low alcohol tolerance
- ☐ Sensitive to loud noises or bright lights
- ☐ Sensitive to wool, heat, cold
- ☐ Sensitive to odors or fragrances
- ☐ Autism, ADHD, or spectrum
- ☐ Feel hungover without drinking alcohol
- ☐ Muscle weakness
- ☐ Multiple confusing symptoms that come and go

Increased Risk

- ☐ History of previous allergies, asthma or other responses listed above
- ☐ Taking antibiotics (now or previously)
- ☐ Taking multiple medications
- ☐ Negative reaction to certain medications (e.g. morphine)
- ☐ Feel worse after taking certain supplements
- ☐ Using toxic chemicals (or exposed to them)
- ☐ Family member has histamine -related issues
- ☐ Hormone imbalance *such as* estrogen dominance
- ☐ Exposed to moldy environment (home, car, school, work)
- ☐ Use plastics for food prep and storage
- ☐ Smoke cigarettes (or related) or exposed to second-hand smoke
- ☐ Consume few fresh fruits and vegetables

- ☐ Consume a lot of sugar or refined carbohydrates (cakes, cookies)
- ☐ High stress
- ☐ Taking painkillers, antacids, steroids, or contraceptive pill
- ☐ Poor diet, fad diet, or restrictive diet
- ☐ Drink alcohol > 1x/week
- ☐ Lack of sleep
- ☐ Late night eating
- ☐ Yeast overgrowth (Candida)
- ☐ Menopause or perimenopause

If you checked:

- **over half** of the boxes in any **one** of the sections, it's **likely** you have excess histamine

- **< 20** boxes on this entire list, it's **unlikely** you have excess histamine

- **20-40** boxes on this entire list, it's **likely** you have excess histamine

- **> 40** of the boxes on this entire list, it's **very likely** you have excess histamine

> *Antibiotics not only inhibit histamine removal but also alter gut bacteria and cause damage to the gut, reducing DAO enzyme production.*

Causes

Simplistically, histamine excess is usually the total load from multiple sources. The chart below shows some of the main histamine contributors.

What Fills Your Histamine Bucket?

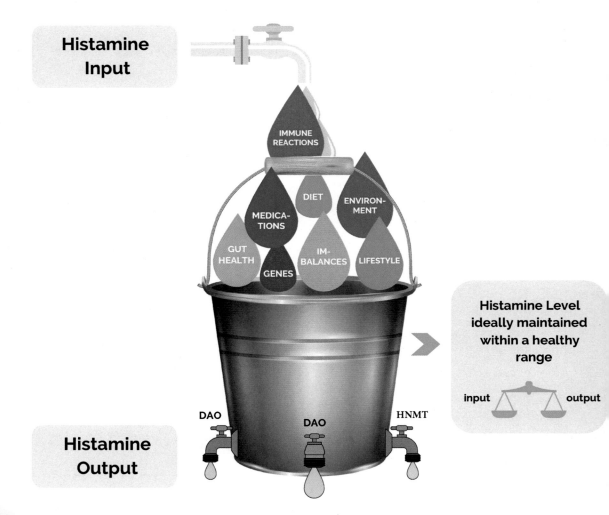

Be mindful of your body.
A reaction is your body's way of telling you something isn't right.

Histamine INPUT is increased by:

- ☐ Diet: intake of high-histamine foods and drinks
- ☐ Certain gut bacterial species that produce histamine
- ☐ Triggers that lead to histamine release from mast cells, such as allergies, infections, artificial dyes, and some medications
- ☐ Natural production of histamine to aid digestion

Histamine OUTPUT is decreased by:

- ☐ Genes: certain changes in genes that code histamine metabolizing enzymes
- ☐ Factors that negatively impact histamine degrading enzymes, such as alcohol and certain medications
- ☐ Gut damage from infections, certain medications such as antibiotics or painkillers or imbalanced gut flora

Testing

First, ruling out more serious conditions such as mastocytosis or acute (IgE-based) allergies is very important.

Second, lab testing isn't definitive for HIT yet but it is rapidly advancing (look out for updates which will be posted on Rider4Health.com.

Thirdly, empirical testing could be more informative. Simply put, if your symptoms are reduced on a low-histamine diet and/or with DAO supplementation, it is not unreasonable to consider HIT as a potential culprit.

Excess histamine can be provoked by a vast number of triggers that lead to diverse symptoms.

Symptoms are often multi-faceted, non-specific, wax and wane, and are often attributed to different diseases.

The good news is that once your histamine levels are rebalanced, your symptoms should start to disappear.

Let's get started! Below are checklists of options, all of which have been shown to help harness histamine levels. Commit to implementing multiple tips in each section. Some will be more relevant to you (bioindividually) and you can refer back to your Self-Test results as a guide. For example, if you checked off more boxes related to **Digestion**, then focus on **digestive solutions** such as those in **Checklist 1, Diet**. However, all the checklists can be helpful.

You can also take clues from your causes or triggers. For example, if you feel that **Stress** is your main trigger, **Checklist 2, Lifestyle** will be important. Or if you feel worse around smokers, fires, mold or other inhaled triggers, then **Checklist 3, Environment** will be important.

You know your body best. Start small and go for slow and steady improvements so you'll be motivated to do more. Prefer the all-or-nothing approach? This plan accommodates you, too. Commit to tackling the options on the Diet, Lifestyle, and Environment checklists, and then incorporate supplements too, if needed.

This information is educational and intended to help support your heath and wellness. It is not a replacement for medical advice.

Many conditions start in the gut. In the case of histamine, this definitely rings true. An unhealthy gut can lead to increased histamine in numerous ways, and what we eat has a direct impact on supporting a healthier gut. In some ways, this is the easiest area to address because it's straightforward. In other ways, it's the most challenging because it's hard to give up the food we love.

As You Go, Keep in Mind

- Histamine Intolerance (HIT) is an indication that you have developed too much histamine, not a sensitivity to histamine itself. This means that rebalancing your histamine level is the goal, not eliminating histamine completely.

- There is an incredibly wide spectrum of histamine reactions from mild issues to chronic or severe reactions. The former group may only need to taper back on the top histamine offenders, whereas the latter may need to be more strict, but not to the point of compromising their nutrient intake.

- Short-term, reducing histamine foods can help lower inflammation, alleviate suffering, and provide a foundation to start healing. ~1-3 weeks is usually effective in my experience.

- Long-term, however, the goal is to heal your root cause and support your overall health.

- Histamine levels in food are often related to the quality, processing, storage method, and age (of the food) rather than the food itself, so choose high quality, unprocessed, very fresh foods. Frozen foods can be just as good if the food was fresh when frozen.

- There are many low histamine diet (LHD) food lists available, but with little consistency. However, the top offenders remain the same and have been used here. Not every possible food has been included to prevent focusing too much on restricting your diet. For links to a longer list, see page 51.

- You will likely also have your own unique dietary trigger(s), regardless of their histamine level, e.g. a specific food allergy. You may already know these or may uncover them through careful diet tracking. Keeping a food log is very helpful! Tracking your lifestyle (e.g. sleep, stress level) as well as environment (e.g. sudden weather or elevation changes, pollen level, cigarette smoke exposure) will all help you understand what is irritating your body's immune system.

- Avoiding blood sugar imbalances by limiting sugary foods is key to healing. Also try to avoid intense hunger which can be stressful to the body.

- While avoiding high histamine foods, first limit foods which are unhealthy (e.g. processed foods) then, if needed, healthy ones. For example, avoid orange juice before oranges.

- Seafood and meats are highly perishable. The longer they are unfrozen, the more histamine they contain. Don't let foods sit out.

- Read food ingredient labels on the back of packages. Artificial dyes, flavors, and preservatives are some of the worst offenders.

Minimize or Avoid These

- ☐ Junk food / Processed foods. Generally, the more processed the food (longer time in the factory) the more inflammatory.
- ☐ Alcohol (especially fermented)
- ☐ Aged cheeses
- ☐ Artificial preservatives (e.g. BHA, BHT, benzoates, sulfites)
- ☐ Artificial dyes (e.g. tartrazine/ FD&C yellow #5, also found in some medications and supplements)
- ☐ Artificial flavors (e.g. MSG or other glutamates)
- ☐ Leftovers, spoiled foods
- ☐ Cured meats (salami, sausage, hot dogs)
- ☐ Pickled foods (e.g. pickles, olives) and some condiments
- ☐ Smoked foods
- ☐ Sugary foods and drinks (sugar feeds unwelcome yeast and bacteria which can cause gut damage)
- ☐ Energy drinks
- ☐ Fermented foods (e.g. sauerkraut, kimchi, kombucha, soy sauce, yogurt)
- ☐ Foods you know give you a reaction such as a specific allergy to peanuts
- ☐ Low-fat diets; go for healthy fats
- ☐ Dehydration (drink plenty of clean water)

- ☐ Cow's milk and products
- ☐ Gluten
- ☐ Fermented teas, black and green
- ☐ Eggplant, spinach, tomatoes and tomato products, avocados
- ☐ Yeast, yeast extracts, and yeast products (e.g. breads, pastries)
- ☐ Dried foods (e.g. prunes, dates)
- ☐ Overripe foods (e.g. squishy avocados)
- ☐ Shellfish
- ☐ Many lists also include the following foods, but reactivity is individual: Citrus, papaya, pineapples, strawberries, raspberries, bananas, soy, potatoes, lentils, beans, some spices, chocolate, cocoa, and some nuts

See the Appendix for a more complete list.

- ☐ Keep a food journal (see blank food logs in the Appendix).

Tracking your diet, lifestyle, environment, supplements, and associated symptoms helps to identify your unique histamine offenders. Be mindful of how your diet affects your body. If you have a reaction, it is likely due to something you ate in the last few hours. However, some symptoms can arise over the next day or two. Carefully keeping track is the most accurate way to pinpoint your triggers. If you discover that you are reacting to a long list of foods, the issue could be more complex, but you can still gain significant benefit from tracking.

Thinking Twice About Giving Up Alcohol?

It can be difficult to give up that relaxing drink at night. But did you know that alcohol:

- Competes for the same metabolic pathway as histamine, meaning they both use the enzyme aldehyde dehydrogenase (ALDH)

- **Contains histamine**
- **Slows down histamine removal**
- **Triggers mast cells**
- **Burdens the liver, which is needed to detox histamine**

Bottom line, alcohol increases histamine.

Foods To Add: Emphasize These For Nutrient-Rich Eating

☐ Fresh, unprocessed foods. For example, choose fresh grapes over raisins.

☐ Whole, fresh veggies and fruits which naturally contain phytonutrients to quench inflammation.

☐ SOUL foods - Seasonal, Organic, Unprocessed, and Local (Dr. Ed Bauman).

☐ Fresh foods, or consider freezing immediately after harvesting or preparing.

☐ Vitamin C rich foods - berries, apples, broccoli, onions, and dandelion greens.

☐ Vitamin B2 rich foods - mushrooms, asparagus, eggs, and almonds.

☐ Vitamin B6 rich foods - cabbage, cauliflower, sweet potato, liver, salmon.

☐ Magnesium-rich foods - leafy greens, almonds and dark chocolate.

☐ Copper rich foods - nuts and seeds, shiitake and crimini mushrooms, if tolerated.

☐ Zinc-rich foods - meats, shellfish (if tolerated), nuts and seeds.

☐ Omega-3 rich foods - wild, cold-water, Frozen-At-Sea (FAS) or very fresh fish such as salmon and halibut. Also freshly-ground flaxseed and chia seeds.

☐ Quality oils - organic, expeller-pressed extra virgin olive oil, avocado oil and coconut oil. Note: Whole avocados may not be tolerated, but the oil is usually tolerated. Remember to store your oils in a dry, cool place away from light. Before you use them, take a whiff and toss any oils with hints of rancidity.

☐ Plenty of other histamine-lowering foods. See the table on the next page and Appendix for more foods.

Strengthen Digestion: Enhance nutrient absorption with strong digestion. Here's how:

☐ Try digestive enzymes just before meals

☐ Chew, chew, chew, and chew

☐ Stimulate digestion by eating dandelion leaves, artichokes, or a squeeze of lemon (if tolerated) in your water before a meal.

☐ Be mindful. Sit down and take it slow when you eat. Rest to digest.

☐ Don't overeat. Stop when you're 80% full.

Eating Habits

☐ Avoid late night eating. Histamine levels peak during the night.

☐ Avoid frying or grilling foods since these methods of cooking may increase histamine levels. Boiling or steaming may be better.

☐ Slow cooking has many health benefits but is not recommended in your early phases of healing due to high histamine levels it can produce. However, you can still enjoy your bone broth if cooked in a pressure cooker for a shorter time (see recipe).

Histamine-Balancing Foods

What	Why	How	Comments
Prebiotics	• Prebiotics feed the probiotics in the gut	• Jerusalem artichoke, garlic, onion, leeks, chicory root, and dandelion greens • Take with probiotics	• Caution if you have digestive upset such as bloating or abdominal pain • Partly indigestible by us, but feed beneficial gut flora
Chamomile	• Inhibits histamine release from masts, dose-dependently	• Enjoy as a relaxing tea	• Caution if you have a ragweed allergy
Ginger	• Good for digestive issues • Mast cell stabilizer	• Slice fresh ginger into small pieces. Add one tablespoon to a cup of water	• Use as tea
Garlic	• Inhibits histamine release	• Chop and let sit 10 mins to activate benefits	• Also a prebiotic. May worsen flatulence in sensitive people
Pea sprouts (*Pisum sativum*)	• DAO enzyme source	• Enjoy whenever, especially with meals	• Grow your own
Turmeric (*Curcumin*)	• Inhibits mast cell activation • Anti-inflammatory • Antioxidant	• Add to soups • Sprinkle on salads, steamed veggies	• Active component of turmeric is curcumin
Watercress (*Nasturtium officinale*)	• Inhibits histamine release from mast cells	• Eat fresh on a sandwich, in a salad or smoothie	• Bitter taste, but worth it
Extra-virgin olive oil (EVOO)	• Anti-inflammatory • Healthy fat	• Use instead of corn, safflower, sunflower, or other commercial seed oils	• Don't cook with high heat. Store in a dark, cool place to prevent oxidation/rancidity
Broccoli sprouts	• Packed with nutrients including sulforaphane, a known histamine reliever	• Eat directly or on salads or sandwiches	• Broccoli also beneficial (You can grow your own)

See more foods in Appendix

Don't underestimate the power of positive lifestyle changes on your health. If you want to get better, take time to take care of yourself — relax, sleep, and breathe. This may sound ridiculously simple, but when all is said and done, it remains a huge challenge for most people. However, it's well worth it and has a huge impact on healing. Stress and lack of sleep lead to raised stress hormones which ultimately adds histamine. On the other hand, when relaxed, the parasympathetic nervous system kicks in and the body naturally digests our food and absorbs nutrients, as well as detoxifies, eliminates, and builds immunity.

Prevention is key. Avoid histamine contributors to lighten the body's workload. Below are tips on how to do this. Remember to think **WESST**:

- [ ] **W**ater: Clean and conveniently placed where you can access and drink it often.
- [ ] **E**xercise but don't overdo it. Think yoga, tai chi, pilates. This is not triathlon time.
- [ ] **S**leep
    - [ ] Sleep in sync with nature's circadian rhythm. Asleep by 10 pm for 7-8 hours.
    - [ ] Avoid blue light at night; it disrupts sleep.
    - [ ] Shut down electronics at least two hours before bed.
    - [ ] Follow a bedtime routine every night.
- [ ] **S**tress less
    - [ ] Try deep breathing into your belly button area.
    - [ ] Try practicing mindfulness, meditation or other peaceful activity daily.
    - [ ] Learn to say no so you don't spread yourself too thin.
    - [ ] Look at your To Do list. What's optional and can be cancelled?
    - [ ] If possible, avoid people and events that stress you out.
    - [ ] Spend quality time with friends.
    - [ ] Turn off the daily news and turn on uplifting media. Better yet, go for a walk and tune into nature.
    - [ ] Take care of yourself. Forgive. Love. Be gentle.
    - [ ] Learn to take things less seriously. Laugh at yourself. Be happy, not perfect.
- [ ] **T**ake care of yourself and your environment
    - [ ] Commit to quit smoking.
    - [ ] Ditch recreational drugs. They slow histamine clearance.
    - [ ] Avoid unnecessary medications, if possible, especially NSAIDs and antibiotics. Note: Speak to your doctor first.
    - [ ] Life happens, but try to reduce your risk of cuts, bug bites, sunburns, burns, and other injuries. These can all add to your histamine bucket.

- ☐ Filter your water
- ☐ Clean your air with a HEPA air filter
- ☐ Ventilate stuffy rooms
- ☐ Remove carpeting and install hardwood floors
- ☐ Use low VOC paints or other chamicals
- ☐ Spend time in nature, or at least more natural places

Nettle leaf

Minimize or Avoid These

- ☐ Mold exposure (thrives in dark and damp areas)
- ☐ Smoking, second hand smoke and other sources of smoke
- ☐ Wildfire smoke, if possible
- ☐ Pesticides such as glyphosate (Roundup)
- ☐ Abrupt changes in temperature or air pressure (e.g. elevation, air travel)
- ☐ Loud noises
- ☐ Bright lights
- ☐ Pollution
- ☐ Harsh chemicals such as bleach
- ☐ High EMF exposure
- ☐ Harsh cleaning and personal care products
- ☐ Dust / dust mites
- ☐ Strong fragrances and odors

Diet, lifestyle, and environment changes are paramount to long-term healing. However, some of us need a little short-term boost from supplements. You see, our food and soil are not as nutrient-rich as they used to be; therefore, no matter how hard we try, it can be difficult to get everything we need from our diet alone — especially if you follow a low-histamine or other restrictive diet.

Histamine-helpful supplements help to lower histamine levels in multiple ways such as supporting histamine-removing enzymes or stabilizing mast cells to prevent histamine release.

Also, with a little help from digestive enzymes we can improve digestion. Lastly, though specific probiotics can boost beneficial bacteria, many are also histamine triggers. That said, those who suffer severe histamine reactivity may do better limiting supplements to start.

The following suggestions have been narrowed down to the most common evidence-based supplements.

Histamine-Balancing Supplements

What	Why	How	Comments
Vitamin C	• Natural Antihistamine • Required for DAO • Anti-inflammatory • Antioxidant	• 250-1000 mg in divided doses • Ascorbyl palmitate form is better than ascorbic acid • Combine with flavonoids for optimal benefit	• Found naturally in berries, apples, broccoli, and leafy greens • May cause loose stool. Start slow and increase to bowel tolerance
Flavonoids, e.g., Rutin, Quercetin, Luteolin, and many others	• Antioxidant • Mast cell stabilizer • Anti-inflammatory • Antioxidant	• 100-500 mg • Combine with vitamin C and other flavonoids for optimal benefit	• Abundant in fresh fruits and vegetables **Quercetin**: apple peel, leafy vegetables, broccoli, grapes **Rutin**: asparagus, apple peel **Luteolin**: celery, thyme, chamomile, broccoli
Vitamin B2	• Required for monoamine oxidase (MAO) enzyme	• 50-100 mg • Active Riboflavin 5' phosphate (R5P) form	• Found in crimini mushrooms, asparagus • Take with B complex supplement to avoid deficiencies

What	Why	How	Comments
Vitamin B6	• Required for DAO enzyme	• 50-100 mg • Active Pyridoxal 5' phosphate (P5P) form	• Found in cabbage, cauliflower, sweet potato, salmon • Take all B vitamins when increasing any one of them long-term
The Right Probiotics	• Help to rebalance the gut microbiota	• Use as directed on supplement label	• Emphasize Histamine-friendly species. Some species worsen histamine symptoms (See Appendix)
Digestive enzymes	• Assists in food digestion • Makes nutrients bioavailable	• Use as directed on supplement label • Take with meals	• Enzyme blends are readily available as supplements • Start with simpler formulations
Omega 3	• Anti-inflammatory • Healthy essential fats	• 1,000-2000 mg • Quality is key; many brands are rancid • Plant sources have lower absorption rates	• Found in fish oil and wild fish such as salmon and halibut. Also, chia and freshly ground flaxseeds. • Choose Frozen-at-Sea (FAS) or very fresh fish
Nettle (Urtica dioica)	• Potent antihistamine • Mast cell stabilizer	• Enjoy as a tea • 400 mg as a supplement	• Some people don't tolerate it well
Holy basil	• Antihistamine • Mast cell stabilizing	• Enjoy as a tea	• Tulsi tea • Fresh basil also helps
Moringa (M. oleifera)	• Antihistamine • Inhibits histamine release	• Add powder to a smoothie or other drink	• Very effective • Start with 1/2 tsp. daily and taper up to avoid diarrhea

What	Why	How	Comments
Butterbur	• Stabilizes mast cells. • Evidence is good, particularly for migraines	• Migraines: Petadolex, 100 mg twice daily for 4-6 months, then taper off. Or whole butterbur root extract (Petaforce) 50 mg twice daily	• Only products labeled "PA-free" should be used • Take supplements short term only (<3-4 months)
Turmeric (Curcumin)	• Inhibits mast cell activation • Anti-inflammatory • Antioxidant	• 500 mg, 1-3 times daily	• Active component of turmeric is curcumin • Supplements with black pepper piperine have better absorbtion
Vitamin D3	• Steroid hormone critically important for immune balancing	• Start with 2000 IU daily to obtain optimal blood levels of 65-75 ug/dl	• The "sunshine" vitamin • Get tested to determine your Vitamin D level • Reduces intestinal inflammation
Multimineral containing copper, iron, and zinc	• Needed for DAO histamine-degrading enzyme (re: copper)	• 2-3 mg daily • Best to get minerals like copper, iron, or zinc from foods (liver, organ meats, almonds, asparagus)	• Supplement with copper or iron **only** if blood tests show deficiencies
Magnesium	• Insufficiency or deficiency is very common • Essential cofactor for hundreds of enzymes and energy production	• 400 - 800 mg. • Leafy greens and Brazil nuts are great sources	• Magnesium supplement taken for too long may deplete calcium • If diarrhea occurs, reduce amount or switch form to magnesium glycinate

What	Why	How	Comments
SAMe	• Supports methylation needed for HNMT enzyme which degrades histamine	• 400-800 mg twice daily	• Don't take with a prescription antidepressant. • Not for Parkinson's patients
DAO enzyme	• Replaces your own DAO enzyme if needed • Main enzyme in the gut that degrades histamine from your diet	• Short-lived, so take immediately before consuming high histamine foods	• If this supplement helps you, insufficient DAO is likely a part of your root issue • DAO doesn't affect histamine elsewhere in the body outside of the gut. • So, if DAO doesn't help you, excess histamine may still be an issue for you, but likely outside the gut

Congratulations!

Now that you're implementing these changes, your histamine levels will be rebalancing. However, it may take days to weeks before you notice consistent benefits.

Friendly Reminders

Track Your Progress: People often don't realize they no longer suffer from, say, itching or brain fog until they look at their progress log (see Appendix). This is yet another reason to track your progress. Also, listen to feedback from your friends, family, and practitioner.

Setbacks Happen: There may be times when you feel a little worse before you feel better. Symptoms are the body's way of dealing with a threat or irritant. Trust that your body is healing itself. Often, we just need to supply our body with nourishment and then get out of its way. Listen to feedback from your body.

Next Steps if You're Not Making Progress

Often-Overlooked Histamine Contributors and Triggers to Avoid

- ☐ Hidden triggers of histamine in foods such as in fancy sauces and dressings
- ☐ Alcohol as a preservative - tinctures
- ☐ Hidden artificial food additives
- ☐ Dyes used in medications
- ☐ Intense exercise
- ☐ Sun exposure. UVB rays can be a histamine trigger
- ☐ Intense heat, cold, or sudden temperature changes
- ☐ Hidden infections - gut or dental
- ☐ Chronic inflammation
- ☐ Air pressure changes - air travel, elevation changes such as ascending mountains
- ☐ Hidden mold in dark, damp, water-damaged areas - bathrooms, basements and front-loading washing machines
- ☐ Eating at restaurants. It's difficult to know ingredients, food quality, or prep methods
- ☐ Low level or yet undiscovered allergies - pets
- ☐ What you wear - wool, nickel jewelry, etc.
- ☐ Physical pressure - a tight ponytail, grinding teeth, etc.

☐ Sensory triggers such as vibrations.

☐ Unrealized sources of stress

☐ Another underlying issue that needs correcting - other deficiencies

This list may seem long, but it is just a sample of the myriad factors that influence histamine levels in the body. Don't worry about every trigger; no one trigger affects every person.

Which factors should you consider avoiding? Some of these are easier to identify as culprits than others. For example, if you're sensitive to wool, you'll likely be very itchy when you wear it.

Step it up. If you are still suffering symptoms of excess histamine at this point, we need to take it up a notch. Here are some higher level suggestions to further reduce histamine overload. It would be prudent to work with a knowledgeable nutritionist / practitioner at this point.

☐ Consider intermittent fasting (I.F.) or time-restricted fasting (TRF). Unlike most fasting, this doesn't limit your calories necessarily, but limits the time of eating to a window. For instance, I often try to eat no later than 6 pm and no earlier than 10 am, to give my digestive system a break for 16 hours. This works well for some people since the simple act of eating triggers histamine release to produce stomach acid to enable digestion. However, fasting for too long can stress your body, exacerbating the problem, so don't overdo it. Also, I.F. is not recommended for everyone, especially children or those who are underweight or with blood sugar dysregulation.

☐ If your symptoms are digestive, such as those of SIBO or IBS, consider a low Fermentable Oligosaccharides, Disaccharides, Monosaccharides, and Polyols (FODMAP) diet. The FODMAP diet is a diet that is used only for a short time, usually 3 to 4 weeks, depending on the person. This is especially useful when someone has digestive symptoms.

For links to more details, see page 51.

☐ Consider a Paleo-like Elimination Diet short-term to help uncover food-based causes and get to the root of the problem. And remember to keep a food log. Simplistically, the Paleo diet includes foods eaten by our ancestors and avoids beans, grains, and dairy. The Elimination diet avoids the 8 major allergens — dairy, eggs, wheat, tree nuts, peanuts, soy, fish, and shellfish — and other major inflammatory foods. After 3-4 weeks, these foods are added back one at a time to test their effect on your body. Do not test foods you know you have an allergy to. For links to more details about this diet, see page 51.

Still No Improvement?

If you did not experience improvement in your histamine symptoms, there could be deeper reasons. Consider the following:

First, you may need longer to notice improvement. Many years of accumulated damage usually takes time to reverse. Committing to a good three to six months without giving up along the way is important.

Second, histamine may not be the only culprit. Although it is an early mediator in inflammation, it is not alone. While reducing histamine levels is helpful for most people, it is not a panacea. Many other inflammatory mediators also impact your health.

Third, there are also more serious conditions of mast cells such as mastocytosis (rare), which can lead to more mast cells and consequently, histamine excess. These possibilities fall outside the scope of this book, in which case I'd highly recommend working with a specialist or mast cell expert to get to the root.

Fourth, you could have a co-existing illness, infection, or sensitivity that is impacting inflammation and therefore histamine levels. I've often seen candida yeast overgrowth in people with persistent histamine excess. So if you do your best to limit histamine foods and still have symptoms, a integrative specialist / practitioner may need to be consulted. Don't try to do this on your own.

Feel free to contact me with questions, comments, feedback. My door is always open!

Rider4health.org

Key Takeaways

☐ Histamine is a powerful little molecule involved in every system of the body and a key mediator in inflammation.

☐ Histamine is necessary but too much can wreak havoc.

☐ Some people have a lower tolerance for histamine, which has been called Histamine Intolerance (HIT).

☐ Symptoms are multifaceted, differ from person to person, range widely from mild to severe, tend to wax and wane, and be unpredictable.

☐ There are acute symptoms such as heartburn as well as delayed or chronic symptoms such as chronic fatigue syndrome.

☐ Underlying causes are also multifaceted, but include gene expression, immune reactions, poor gut health, imbalances in nutrients, hormone imbalances, diet, lifestyle, environment, and medications.

☐ Various low histamine food lists exist but vary considerably, except for the top offenders.

☐ A low histamine diet (LHD) is a short term fix. Healing the root cause should be the focus.

☐ Rebalancing histamine for recovery can be based on your specific causes (if known) and involve implementing changes from the checklists in this book.

I've seen numerous people rebalance their histamine levels and return to feeling revitalized. This is what I hope for you too!

Frequently Asked Questions (FAQ)

Why are my symptoms so different from my sister's?

For one, there are different histamine receptors throughout the body leading to different reactions. You may be familiar with some of the medications that block these. Antihistamines such as Zyrtec, Claritin, and Allegra block one histamine receptor to reduce allergy symptoms, while Antacids such as Pepcid, Tagamet, Axid and Zantac block another histamine receptor to reduce stomach upset/reflux..

Second, there are four kinds of histamine receptors on cells, numbered 1 through 4, and different kinds of cells have different histamine receptors. Differences in how those receptors are expressed from one person to another may help account for why some people get headaches, others GI problems, etc.

Why Doesn't My Doctor Know About Histamine Intolerance?

Your doctor may act perplexed if you say "Histamine Intolerance" First, it's not an actual medical diagnosis but a colloquial term used to describe patterns of symptoms that may seem unrelated to a non-immunologist.

In fact, the medical profession has been addressing histamine effects on different systems since 1942 when Bernard N. Halpern created the first antihistamine, a histamine receptor 1 (H1R) blocker for hay fever and runny nose. And by the late 1970s, blockers of histamine receptor 2 (H2R) were used for peptic ulcers. You may even have been prescribed some of these antacids or gastrointestinal medications: Pepcid, Tagamet, Zantac, and Axid.

H3R and H4R blockers, created in 1987 and 1999 respectively, are being trialed for use with obesity, memory issues, learning deficits, epilepsy and asthma. The bottom line is that HIT is not a term used in formal diagnosis.

Why do I feel so much worse with my monthly period?

Mast cells have estrogen receptors, so estrogen can impact mast cell activation and subsequent release of histamine. This means your symptoms may flare when your estrogen levels are higher compared to your other hormone levels, typically around the time of ovulation (days 11 to 14 of your cycle) as well as just before your menses. The balance or the ratio of estrogen to progesterone is important.

Tips for balancing hormones include avoiding plastics (e.g. BPA, which is a xenoestrogen and interferes with the estrogen pathway), optimizing your weight, exercising, avoiding

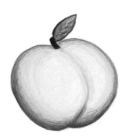

hormone-containing foods such as commercial meats and dairy, increasing dietary fiber, and enjoying hormone-optimizing foods such as beets, carrots, onions, artichokes, dandelion greens, radishes, broccoli, cauliflower and other cruciferous vegetables.

Why does excess histamine make me so drippy?

Think of histamine as a method to purge unwanted substances from your body. For example, if you breathe in pollen, you could sneeze with the goal of expelling it.

Likewise, symptoms such as a runny nose, watery eyes, coughing, vomiting, and diarrhea are methods to expel what the body deems as potentially dangerous. Excess salivation and sweating, as well as rashes could also be included.

For links to more FAQs, see page 51.

Appendix

1. Histamine-Helpful Foods
2. Histamine UNhelpful Foods
3. Histamine-Helpful Probiotics
4. Histamine-UNhelpful Probiotics
5. Medications That Inhibit DAO or Increase Histamine
6. Food Log
7. Symptoms Log
8. Glossary
9. References and Resources
10. Recipes

1. Histamine-Helpful Foods

Fruits (avoid dried, overripe, processed)

- [ ] Apples
- [ ] Apricots
- [ ] Asian pears
- [ ] Blackberries
- [ ] Blueberries
- [ ] Cantaloupe
- [ ] Cherries
- [ ] Coconut
- [ ] Cranberries
- [ ] Fig
- [ ] Goji berry
- [ ] Grapes
- [ ] Honeydew
- [ ] Longans
- [ ] Lychee
- [ ] * Mango
- [ ] Mangosteen
- [ ] Melon
- [ ] Nectarine
- [ ] Passion Fruit
- [ ] Peaches
- [ ] Pears
- [ ] Persimmon
- [ ] Plantain
- [ ] Pomegranate
- [ ] Quince
- [ ] Star Fruit
- [ ] Watermelon

Veggies (avoid dried, overripe, processed)

- [ ] Artichoke
- [ ] Arugula
- [ ] Asparagus
- [ ] Beets
- [ ] Bok choy
- [ ] Broccoli
- [ ] Brussel sprouts
- [ ] Cabbage
- [ ] Cauliflower
- [ ] Carrots
- [ ] Celery
- [ ] Collard
- [ ] Cucumber
- [ ] Endive
- [ ] * Garlic
- [ ] * Green Peas
- [ ] Green leafy vegetables
- [ ] Jicama
- [ ] Kale
- [ ] Kohlrabi
- [ ] Leeks
- [ ] Lettuces (various)
- [ ] * Potatoes
- [ ] Okra
- [ ] * Onion / Shallots
- [ ] Parsnips
- [ ] Radishes
- [ ] Rutabaga
- [ ] * Snow / snap peas
- [ ] Sprouts (any kind)
- [ ] Squashes
- [ ] Sweet Potatoes
- [ ] Turnips
- [ ] Watercress
- [ ] Yams
- [ ] Zucchini

Herbs and More

- [ ] Basil
- [ ] Chamomile
- [ ] Cilantro
- [ ] Dill
- [ ] Fennel
- [ ] Ginger
- [ ] Holy Basil
- [ ] Mint / Peppermint
- [ ] Moringa
- [ ] Parsley
- [ ] Pea Sprouts
- [ ] Rosemary
- [ ] Sage
- [ ] Tarragon
- [ ] Thyme
- [ ] Turmeric

Meat/Fish/Protein (must be fresh or frozen)

- [ ] *Almond butter
- [ ] Beef
- [ ] Chicken
- [ ] Duck
- [ ] Goose
- [ ] Cooked eggs
- [ ] Turkey
- [ ] Freshly-caught or Frozen-At-Sea (FAS) Fish

> * Particularly sensitive people may still react or react more strongly to these foods; use caution

Fats/Oils

Most cold-pressed oils, such as extra virgin olive oil, coconut oil, flaxseed oil, and avocado oil. (Note: avoid processed oils containing preservatives such as BHA and BHT.)

Grains/Nuts/Seeds

- [ ] Amaranth
- [ ] Chia
- [ ] Flax Seeds
- [ ] Oats (gluten-free)
- [ ] Hemp seeds
- [ ] Millet
- [ ] Quinoa
- [ ] Rice
- [ ] Sorghum
- [ ] Macadamia nuts
- [ ] Chestnuts
- [ ] Rice noodles

Other

- [ ] Baking powder & soda
- [ ] Coconut sugar
- [ ] Crackers without yeast or artificial ingredients
- [ ] Sea salt, unrefined
- [ ] Coconut milk
- [ ] Some herbal teas
- [ ] Honey
- [ ] Maple syrup
- [ ] Rice milk
- [ ] Organic coffee
- [ ] Stevia
- [ ] Pure jams made with allowed ingredients
- [ ] Pure, unbleached flour from allowed foods

2. Histamine-UNhelpful Foods

Additives

- * Alcohol (beer, champagne, wine)
- * Processed foods
- * Any ingredient with glutamate, glutamic acid
- (MSG)
- * Benzoate, benzoic acid
- Alginate
- * Iodide, iodine
- Sobates, sorbic acid
- Sulfur, sulfites
- Carrageenan
- Carmine
- Carmoisine
- Quinine (e.g. tonic water)
- * Food dyes (esp. Yellow, Red, Black)
- Licorice
- Annatto
- BHA, BHT
- and many more

Fruits and Veggies

- Citrus (oranges, mandarins, limes)
- Papaya
- Banana
- Dried fruits
- (prunes, dates)
- Coconut flakes
- Some trail mixes
- Tomatoes
- Tomato sauces
- Eggplant
- Spinach
- Avocado
- Pickles
- Pickled veggies
- Olives
- *Sauerkraut
- Kimchi
- Vinegared veggies

Herbs and More

- * Soy sauce
- * Fish sauce
- Vinegar, wine, balsamic
- * Yeast extract
- Bouillon
- Cumin
- Mustard seeds
- Fenugreek
- Cocoa
- Carob
- Algae and derivatives
- Seaweeds (kelp, kombu, nori, wakame)
- Ketchup
- Relish
- Mustard
- Dressing and sauces with multiple confusing ingredients

Meat/Fish/Protein

- Anchovies, sardines, tuna
- Bone broth
- Smoked fish
- Smoked meats
- Dried meat (jerky)
- Ham (dried or cured)
- Hotdogs
- Sausages (all kinds)
- Salami / Pepperoni
- Soy / tofu
- Crab
- Crayfish
- Lobster
- Oysters
- Clams
- Mussels
- Shrimp
- Raw egg white
- * Cheese (aged, blue, or mold)
- Processed cheese
- Ready-made cheeses
- Pickled fish and meats

Grains/Nuts/Seeds

- Buckwheat
- Sunflower seeds
- Wheat germ
- Peanuts
- Gluten (wheat, rye, barley, spelt, etc.)
- Walnuts

Everyone is unique, and specific foods from the helpful list—while okay for most people—may not be optimal for you and may lead to more histamine. For example, in the case of small intestine bacterial overgrowth (SIBO), some of these foods can worsen bloating, in which case a low-FODMAP diet would be recommended. For links to more recommendations, see page 51.

Other

- Any product past the expiry dates
- Soy milk
- Soda drinks (Coke, Pepsi)
- Hot chocolate
- Kombucha
- Gummy supplements
- Low-quality supplements

3. Histamine-Helpful Probiotics

- *Bifidobacterium longum*
- *Bifidobacterium infantis*
- *Bifidobacterium lactis*
- *Bifidobacterium bifidum*
- *Bifidobacterium breve*
- *Lactobacillus plantarum*
- *Lactobacillus gasseri*
- *Lactobacillus salivarius*
- *Lactobacillus sporogenes*
- Some Soil-based organisms (SBO's)

4. Histamine-UNhelpful Probiotics

- *Lactobacillus delbrueckii*
- *Lactobacillus bulgaricus*
- *Lactobacillus helveticus*
- *Lactobacillus reuteri*
- *Lactobacillus fermentum*
- *Streptococcus thermophilus*

5. Medications That Inhibit DAO or Increase Histamine

Antibiotics
- Cefuroxime (Ceftin)
- Cefotiam (Pansporin)
- Isoniazid, (Hyzyd) used to treat TB
- Pentamidine, an antifungal
- Ciprofloxacin
- Chloroquine (Aralen), an antimalarial

Muscle Relaxants
- Pancuronium (Pavulon)
- Alcuronium (Robaxin)
- D-tubocurarine (Tubocurarine)

Narcotics (barbiturates)
- Thiopental, for relaxation before general anesthesia

Heart Medications
- Dobutamine, congestive heart failure
- Propafenone (Rythmol), heart rhythm

Painkillers
- Morphine
- NSAIDs – Ibuprofen (Advil, Motrin), Naproxen (Aleve), Celecoxib (Celebrex)
- Acetylsalicylic acid (Aspirin)
- Meperidine (Demerol)
- Prilocaine (Lidocaine)

Mental Health
- Amitriptyline (Elavil)
- Diazepam (Valium)
- Haloperidol (Haldol)

Antacids
- Cimetidine (Tagamet)
- Ranitdine (Zantac)

Anti-Asthmatic/Lung Function
- Acetylcysteine (Mucomyst)
- Ambroxol

Blood Pressure Lowering
- Verapamil
- Alprenolol
- Hydralazine

Diuretic
- Amiloride (Midamor)

GI / Vomiting
- Metoclopramide (Reglan)

Other
- Heparin, blood thinner
- Imaging contrast media
- Cyclophosphamide

(Modified from Joneja, J. 2017)

6. Food Log

Keep daily track of everything you consume and your symptoms

FOOD/DRINK	MEDS & SUPPLEMENTS	HOW DID YOU FEEL BEFORE?	HOW DID YOU FEEL AFTER?

7. Symptoms Log

If you experience symptoms, try to recall everything you ate and drank

DATE	SYMPTOMS	WHAT YOU JUST ATE?	WHAT YOU ATE TODAY?	WHAT YOU ATE YESTERDAY?

Contact Dermatitis

Skin inflammation caused by contact with various chemical, animal or plant substances. The reaction may be either a specific immune response or a direct toxic effect of the substance (e.g., poison ivy). The usual suspects include laundry detergent, nickel (in jewelry, zips, and other fastenings), chemicals in rubber gloves, certain cosmetics, certain plants, and topical medications.

DAO Inhibitors

Substances that have a negative effect on DAO enzyme production and/or activity and therefore slow histamine removal. These include many medications, and alcohol, and should be avoided when possible.

Diamine Oxidase (DAO) Enzyme

The enzyme that breaks down histamine extracellularly, or on the outside of the body's cells. It's produced in the lining of the gut and is the main enzyme that degrades histamine ingested from the diet.

Eczema

A skin inflammation, which causes itching and sometimes crusting, scaling or blisters. "Atopic dermatitis" is a type of eczema often made worse by allergens.

Histamine-N-methyltransferase (HNMT) Enzyme

The enzyme responsible for degrading histamine on the inside of cells, in contrast to the enzyme DAO which degrades histamine on the outside of cells. HNMT assists the transfer of a methyl group from S-adenosylmethionine (SAMe), for example, onto histamine. The resulting compound, N-methyl-histamine, is then excreted.

Histamine Decarboxylase (HDC) Enzyme

The only enzyme needed in the body to make histamine from the amino acid histidine, which is found in many foods, particularly foods containing protein. HDC is produced by mast cells and even some bacteria.

Histamine Liberators/Releasers

Substances that can activate mast cells causing release of histamine and other mediators. These include medications (actives as well as additives), and mold, and should be avoided when possible.

Hives

An allergic skin condition, also known as urticaria, characterized by itchy, raised bumps surrounded by an area of red inflammation.

Immune System

A collection of cells and proteins that work together in complex ways to protect the body from potential harm, but also drives histamine intolerance, mast cell disorders, allergies, and hypersensitivities.

Immunoglobulins (Ig's)

Proteins that function as antibodies, such as Immunoglobulin G (IgG) and Immunoglobulin E (IgE). They are produced by immune cells called B-lymphocytes. Their function is to bind to substances in the body that are recognized as foreign (e.g., the surface of bacteria). Ig's also play a central role in allergies when they bind to harmless allergens and provoke histamine release from mast cells.

Inflammation

A complex process characterized by tissue redness, swelling, heat and pain due to injury or infection. It occurs during allergic reactions in the nose, lungs, and skin.

Lymphocyte

A type of white blood cell (WBC) crucially important to the adaptive part of the body's immune system. Lymphocytes mount a specific, tailor-made defense when they detect danger.

Mast Cell

A type of white blood cell important in first line immune defense and central to allergy-type reactions. Mast cells reside in most if not all tissues, mainly located in areas that come into contact with the external environment such as the gut, skin, mouth and lungs. They produce and store histamine and multiple other powerful mediators, ready to rapidly release their arsenal upon provocation.

Mast Cell Activation

A change in mast cell behavior that occurs after exposure to a trigger that may indicate allergy or infection; a state in which mast cells release mediators; in some instances, culminating in anaphylaxis.

Mast Cell Activation Syndrome (MCAS)

A mast cell disease caused by overactive, malfunctioning mast cells, not high numbers of mast cells or an infection. The mast cells release chemical mediators called degranulators that trigger negative effects, such as an immune system response. One of the chemical mediators is histamine, which can lead to an excess of histamine.

Mast Cell Stabilizers

Substances, including medications, that prevent the release of mast cell mediators, such as histamine, through stabilization of the mast cell membrane. These stabilizers are most effective when used prior to trigger exposure.

Mastocytosis

A rare condition characterized by a greater number of mast cells that accumulate in skin and organs. It is usually caused by genetic mutations.

Mediator

A substance released from a cell that affects the environment outside the cell. Examples of mast cell mediators include histamine and tryptase.

Rhinitis

An inflammation of the mucous membrane that lines the nose, often due to an allergy to pollen, dust or other airborne substances. Seasonal rhinitis, aka "hay fever," causes sneezing, itching, a runny nose and nasal congestion.

SNPs (Single nucleotide polymorphisms)

Variations in a single base pair of a gene that can affect the production and/or activity of that gene's product. For example, the gene for the HNMT enzyme could have one of 11 different SNPs, which affects how efficiently the body degrades histamine.

9. References and Resources

Afrin, LB. (2016). *Never Bet Against OCCAM.* Sisters Media, LLC, Bethesda MD.

Afrin LB et al. (2017). *Characterization of mast cell activation syndrome.* Am J Med Sci. 353(3), 207

Afrin LB et al. (2016). *Often seen, rarely recognized: mast cell activation disease–a guide to diagnosis and therapeutic options. Annals of Medicine.* 48(3),190

Bauman, E., et al. (2015). *Therapeutic Nutrition* (Part 1 & 2). Bauman College.

Burkhart, A. *Histamine Intolerance-Could It Be Causing Your Symptoms?* Retrieved from: https://theceliacmd.com/articles/histamine-intolerance-causing-symptoms/. Accessed Sept. 3, 2019.

Carnahan, J. *Mold is a major trigger of mast activation cell syndrome.* https://www.jillcarnahan.com/2018/03/12/mold-is-a-major-trigger-of-mast-activation-cell-syndrome/ Accessed Sept. 3, 2019.

Carnahan, J. *Archives: histamine.* https://www.jillcarnahan.com/tag/histamine/ Accessed Sept. 3, 2019.

Chung, B., et al. (2017) *Effect of different cooking methods on histamine levels in selected foods.* Ann Dermatol. 706-714.

Gershon, M. (1998). *The Second Brain: The Scientific Basis of Gut Instinct and a Groundbreaking New Understanding of Nervous Disorders of the Stomach and Intestines.* New York, NY: Harper.

Jarisch, R. (2015). *Histamine Intolerance: Histamine and Seasickness.* Springer-Verlag Berlin Heidelberg.

Joneja, J. (2003). *Dealing With Food Allergies.* Bull Publishing Company.

Joneja, J. (2017). *Histamine Intolerance: The Complete Guide for Healthcare Professionals.* Berrydales Books.

Joneja, J. (2009). *Histamine Intolerance. It looks like allergy; feels like allergy, but it's not allergy.* J. Action Against Allergy. 97:7-15

Jung, K., et al. (2016). *Contributions of microbiome and mechanical deformation to intestinal bacterial overgrowth and inflammation in a human gut-on-a-chip.* Proceeding of the National Academy of Sciences USA, 113(1).

Karr, T. (2018). *Our Journey with Food*, 2nd Edition. Summerland Publishing.

Kovacova-Hanuskova, E., et al. (2015). *Histamine, Histamine intoxication and intolerance.* Allergol Immunopathol (Madr.) 43(5): 498-506.

Kresser, C. (2019). RHR: *What you should know about histamine intolerance.* https://chriskresser.com/what-you-should-know-about-histamine-intolerance/

Kresser, C. (2019). *Could your histamine intolerance really be mast cell activation disorder?* https://chriskresser.com/could-your-histamine-intolerance-really-be-mast-cell-activation-disorder/

Kresser, C. (2019). *Headaches, hives and heartburn: Could histamine be the cause?* https://chriskresser.com/headaches-hives-and-heartburn-could-histamine-be-the-cause/

Lynch, B. (2018). *Dirty Genes: A Breakthrough Program to Treat the Root Cause of Illness and Optimize Your Health.* New York, New York: HarperCollins.

Maintz L., et al. (2007). *Histamine and histamine intolerance.* Am J Clin Nutr;85(5):1185.

Masini, E., et al. (2007). "*Pea seedling histaminase as a novel therapeutic approach to anaphylactic and inflammatory disorders. A plant histaminase in allergic asthma and ischemic shock.*" Scientific World Journal, 7:888-902.

Matthews, J. (2019). *When histamine goes haywire. Histamine and mast cell activation syndrome – everything you need to know* https://bioindividualnutrition.com/when-histamine-goes-haywire Accessed Sept. 1, 2019.

Pfeiffer, C. (1988). *Nutrition and Mental Illness: An Orthomolecular Approach to Balancing Body Chemistry.* Simon & Schuster, 1988.

Pongdee, T. (2011). *Food Allergy Vs. Food Intolerance.* https://www.aaaai.org/Aaaai/media/MediaLibrary/PDF%20Documents/Libraries/EL-food-allergies-vs-intolerance-patient.pdf

Ruscio, M. (2018). Healthy Gut, Healthy You. The Ruscio Institute LLC.

Ruscio, M. Dr. Ruscio Radio: *Health, Nutrition and Functional Medicine Podcasts.* https://podcasts.apple.com/us/podcast/dr-ruscio-radio-health-nutrition-and-functional-medicine/id983386815 Accessed August 2019.

Science Daily (2019). *Parasympathetic Nervous System.* Retrieved from: https://www.sciencedaily.com/terms/parasympathetic_nervous_system.htm. Sept. 12, 2019.

Swiss Interest Group Histamine Intolerance (SIGHI). https://www.histaminintoleranz.ch/en/introduction.html Accessed Sept. 5, 2019.

Theoharides, TC. (2015). *Mast Cell Disorders.* Blog Talk Radio. https://www.blogtalkradio.com/thecoffeeklatch/2015/02/04/dr-theoharides--mast-cell-disorders-1. Accessed Aug 2019.

Theoharides, TC. (2015). *Mast Cell Disorders.* https://www.mastcellmaster.com/research.php Accessed Aug 2019.

Vickery, A. *Histamine and estrogen.* (2016). Alison Vickery, Holistic Health Coach. https://alisonvickery.com.au/estrogen/. Accessed Sept. 9, 2019.

Wohrl, H. et al. (2004). *Histamine intolerance-like symptoms in healthy volunteers after oral provocation with liquid histamine. Allergy Asthma Proc. 25;5.*

Zimatkin, SM. et al. (1999). *Alcohol-histamine interactions.* Alcohol and Alcoholism;34(2):141-7.

10. Recipes

Apple Oatmeal

Yield: 4 serving; time: 40 minutes

Ingredients:
1 Organic apple
1 cup gluten free, steel cut oatmeal (Irish oats)
4 cups water, filtered preferred
Organic pastured butter
Real maple syrup

Directions:
1. Cut the apple into small chunks.
2. Boil water on high in a medium-sized pot on the stove.
3. Sprinkle the oatmeal into the boiling water. Stir until smooth and starting to thicken.
4. Cook on medium heat for 30 minutes, stirring occasionally.
5. Add 1 teaspoon of real maple syrup and serve.

Note: Irish oats are different than regular oats. The Irish oats have to be cooked longer and need twice as much water to soften them. For example, 1 cup oats will rehydrate with 2 cups water, while Irish oats needs 4 cups water. You can still use regular oats in this recipe but simply use half the water.

Sweet Potato Bites

Yield: 4 servings; time: 40 minutes

Ingredients:
2-4 sweet potatoes, cut into shoestrings
Avocado oil or coconut oil
Sea salt to taste

Directions:
1. Preheat oven to 425° F.
2. Oil small to medium baking dish.
3. Scrub and dry sweet potatoes.
4. Slice sweet potatoes into 2-inch chunks or shoestrings.
5. Drizzle with oil and sprinkle with salt. Place on baking dish.
6. Bake for 30-35 minutes and test for doneness. Bake for an additional 5 minutes or until done.

Apple Beet Arugula Salad

Yield: 4 servings; time: 40 minutes

Ingredients:
1-2 organic apples
3 organic red beets. (Alternatively, use 1 package of pre-cooked organic beets. The brand "Love Beets" is popular.)
4-6 oz (or 2 loose handfuls) organic baby arugula
1-2 cups organic goat cheese crumbles
1-3 tablespoons extra virgin olive oil

Directions:
1. Trim the tops off the beets and steam with skin on until fork tender, about 30 minutes.
2. Allow beets to cool and peel.
3. Chop the beets and the apples into medium-sized chunks. Place them into a medium-sized bowl.
4. Add olive oil. Toss.
5. Add goat cheese crumbles to taste and tolerance level.
6. Mix ingredients together and then add arugula.
7. Serve this delish salad.

Cilantro-Dusted Pork Chops

Yield: 4 servings

Ingredients:
1 pork chop, ½ inch thick
1 tablespoon grass-fed butter
Salt and pepper
5 or so thin lemon slices
1 tablespoon lemon juice
3 cloves of garlic, minced
Cilantro, minced

Directions:
1. Preheat oven to 375° F.
2. Heat oven-proof pan on high.
3. Season pork chop generously with salt and pepper.
4. Add butter to pan until foamy.
5. Put in pork chops and brown on one side for 2-3 minutes.

6. Turn over to sear other side, and add garlic, lemon slices, and lemon juice to the pan.
7. As pork browns, spoon the lemon garlic mixture over the pork.
8. Transfer pork to oven to cook until internal temperature reaches 145-150° F (time can range from 5-25 minutes depending on the thickness of pork chop).
9. Let rest 5 minutes before serving.
10. Sprinkle with cilantro.

Roasted Carrots and Parsnips

Yield: 2-4 servings; time: 30 minutes

Ingredients:
3 carrots, peeled and sliced into 1-inch chunks
3 parsnips, peeled and sliced into 1-inch chunks
2 tablespoons avocado oil or coconut oil
Salt and pepper to taste
1 tablespoon fresh oregano, finely chopped

Directions:
1. Preheat oven to 425° F.
2. Add parchment paper to a sheet tray.
3. Toss carrots and parsnips with oil, salt, pepper and oregano.
4. Place carrots and parsnips on the lined sheet tray.
5. Roast for 12 minutes. Turn carrots and parsnips to cook other side.
6. Roast for another 12-15 minutes until done.

Roasted Asparagus

Yield: 4 servings; time: 25 minutes

Ingredients:
1 bunch of asparagus
Avocado oil or coconut oil
Salt and pepper

Directions:
1. Preheat oven to 425° F.
2. Add parchment paper to a sheet tray.
3. Wash and dry asparagus, and break off ends.
4. Pour oil over asparagus and roll around until covered.
5. Sprinkle salt and pepper to meet your tastes.
6. Bake for 7 minutes. Test for doneness. If not tender enough, bake for additional 3-5 minutes.

Ginger Chicken

Yield: 2 servings; time: 50 minutes

Ingredients:
2 bone-in, skin on chicken breasts
Salt and pepper
1 tablespoon avocado oil or coconut oil
1 inch fresh ginger, peeled and minced
1 garlic clove, minced
2 teaspoons apple cider vinegar
2 tablespoon lemon juice
2/3 cup water
1 tablespoon honey

Directions:
1. Preheat oven to 425° F.
2. Season chicken with salt and pepper.
3. Put chicken in oven for 30-40 minutes, or until internal temperature of 165 degrees.
4. Heat oil in skillet over medium heat.
5. Toss in ginger and garlic and saute for 2 minutes.
6. Add in apple cider vinegar, lemon juice, water and honey.
7. Bring to a boil, then reduce to simmer until sauce thickens (2-3 minutes).
8. Cut chicken up into bite-sized pieces. Pour the pan sauce over chicken. Enjoy!

Low-Histamine Bone Broth

Yield: 2+ quarts. Time: 4-1/4 hours

Very fresh meat is one of the big keys to a low-histamine bone broth. The meat could be chicken wings or beef marrow bones. Ask your butcher how fresh the meat is that you are purchasing, and if there are there any additives. The fresher the meat is, the lower the histamine content. Don't settle for wings or marrow that is older than three or four days, as the bacteria on these foods create histamine. If you can get exceptionally fresh meat, you are as good as gold. And then go home and start the recipe immediately.

Ingredients
1-1/2 lbs beef marrow bones or 2-1/2 lbs chicken wings with skin
1 leek, sliced
2 long carrots, cut in chunks
1 parsnip, cut in chunks
1 cup sliced celery
2 white onions (lower in histamine than yellow onions), diced
1 tablespoon olive oil

1 bunch parsley
1 tablespoon sage
1 tablespoon fresh rosemary
1 tablespoon thyme, preferably fresh
1 tablespoon fresh oregano
Garlic (if tolerated)
Black pepper to taste
Sea salt to taste
1 tablespoon apple cider vinegar or lemon juice (if tolerated) (Pulls out minerals from the bones)
2 quarts water

Stovetop Cooking Directions:

1. In a large soup pot, add the olive oil and onions. Saute until translucent.
2. Next add about half the chicken wings. Brown them; this will give you good color and flavor for the broth.
3. Now it's time to add the rest of the chicken wings, vegetables and all the herbs/spices, including salt and pepper.
4. Fill the pot with water at least two-thirds full. Then add the apple cider vinegar and/or lemon.
5. Turn burner on medium-high and cover pot. Once broth boils, turn down the heat to low.
6. Simmer for 4 hours. Check the broth at least once an hour and remove any scum that forms at the top.
7. Let broth cool slightly before straining.
8. Transfer the strained mixture to containers. Cool before freezing.
9. Note that the fat will rise to the top of the container. This is like a natural preservative so leave it intact until you first open the container for use. If you prefer less fat, remove the fat after opening.

Pressure Cooker Directions:

1. Add all ingredients to pressure cooker, including water.
2. Turn pressure cooker to high heat until pressure builds up.
3. Then turn heat to medium.
4. Cook for two hours.
5. Strain broth and serve or freeze after it cools. Freezing the broth in ice cube trays makes it easy to use the broth daily or in various recipes.

Healthy Endings: David, Amanda and Betty

In the Introduction, some case histories about people suffering from Histamine Intolerance were told. Now you need a follow-up.

David was the one with the allergies. He wasn't willing to change his diet too much, but changed jobs, removing himself from a stressful work environment – one that likely had high electromagnetic fields (EMFs) from computers and wireless technology; high EMFs can exacerbate histamine and stress hormones in the body.

David's runny nose and itchy, watery, and reddened eyes subsided, illustrating how sometimes a lifestyle change could be all that's needed to ease symptoms. He doesn't use antihistamines much anymore. He reported that he's much healthier now, too. Obtaining a good night's sleep is his last challenge, but at least he is not waking up at night due to congestion.

Amanda was the one who had migraines that ruined her quality of life. It wasn't enough to change her diet to mostly healthy foods; what could be wrong?

Her A-ha moment came when she noticed a pattern on her daily food log. While trying to eat healthier, she had been emphasizing bone broth, fermented foods, yogurt, spinach, avocados, protein powers, and the wrong probiotics. Who knew that something as good as kombucha could be bad for anyone?

"Mainly I worked on getting my gut right. Once I started, my symptoms were like night and day – within only a few days," Amanda stated. "and I have far fewer migraines."

"I know when I've over-indulged at a wine and cheese or beer and pizza party. I wake up feeling hungover. Even my eyeballs feel fat." Amanda also discovered she had a mutation in the HNMT gene. As mentioned earlier, both HNMT and DAO are vital for histamine removal.

Betty was the teacher with terrible digestive symptoms. She had been diagnosed with SIBO. This called for a total recolonization of her gut. She added histamine-friendly probiotics for gut healing and followed a low FODMAP diet. However, the diet wasn't enough, so after two months, she focused on low-histamine foods. Lab testing uncovered a severe anemia and vitamin D deficiency that was addressed as well.

At the last check-in with Betty before she moved out of the area, she had regained weight lost and reported that most of her symptoms were better. She didn't look like she was pregnant anymore; her bloating had mostly subsided.

◇◇◇◇◇◇◇◇◇◇◇◇◇◇◇◇◇◇◇◇◇◇◇◇◇◇

As for Tayla, the inspiration of this book (and my life), the little girl mentioned in "My Story," she is thriving. The only time she doesn't feel good is when she overindulges at a Halloween party or other candy-fest. Then, for the next few days she has a general unwellness that's difficult to describe — headaches, stomachaches, fatigue, brain fog, dark circles under her eyes — almost like she's hungover. Sometimes she becomes anxious, moody, and seemingly more susceptible to illnesses during this time. Some of these symptoms could be due to a yeast overgrowth, fueled by the excess sugar. The yeast Candida is known to trigger mast cells, adding to histamine levels.

Overall, she has made so much progress in her health journey, and it's a real blessing to her mother (me!) to watch her grow up. Over the years I've done what I can to help Tayla and many clients like her. And after years of research and trial and error, I've found the tips outlined in this book to be the most helpful to heal the histamine hangover.

◇◇

These are some of the many histamine stories with healthy endings, and I hope they give you hope. Excess histamine can be harnessed!

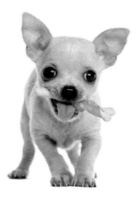

And the Chihuahua (mast cell) is peaceful again.

The End

Website specific to this book:
Rider4Health.org

An online symptoms survey:
bit.ly/2U191dP

Made in the USA
Monee, IL
11 November 2022

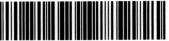

17531742R00036